DASH DIET COOKB

FOR BEGINNERS

21-Day Dash Diet Meal Plan to Lose Weight and Lower Your Blood Pressure

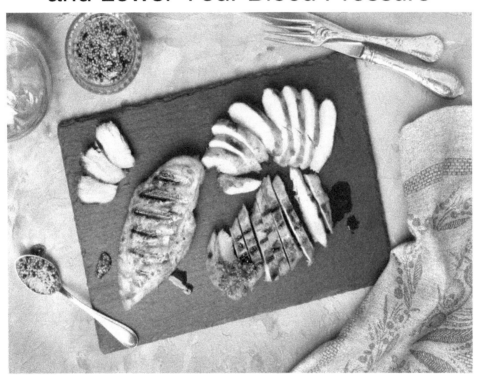

Table of Contents

BREAKFAST RECIPES

LUNCH RECIPES

Classic Chicken Noodle Soup

DINNER RECIPES

Fennel Sauce Tenderloin

Beefy Fennel Stew

Currant Pork Chops

Spicy Tomato Shrimp

Beef Stir Fry

Shrimp & Corn Chowder

Leek & Cauliflower Soup

Easy Beef Brisket

Coconut Shrimp

Asian Salmon

Basil Halibut

SIDE DISH RECIPES

Pesto Mushrooms

Lemon Green Beans with Almonds

Sweet & Savory Brussel Sprouts

Caramelized Sweet Potatoes

Vegetable & Polenta Dish

Rosemary Potato Skins

Squash Fries

Vegetable Kebabs

DESSERT RECIPES

Toasted Almond Ambrosia

Apple Dumplings

Apricot Biscotti

Apple & Berry Cobbler

Mixed Fruit Compote Cups

Oatmeal Surprise Cookies

CONCLUSION

INTRODUCTION

Before we get into our 21-day meal plan and DASH diet guide, let's look at what the Dash Diet stands for. "Dietary Approaches to Stop Hypertension" is what it means, so as the name suggest it's meant to control hypertension through the way you eat. It's a common misconception that this means you'll be on a vegetarian diet, but it's a well-balanced diet that mainly focuses on low fat dairy, fruits, whole grains and vegetables. You minimize fat and sodium, but that doesn't mean you have to cut meat out completely.

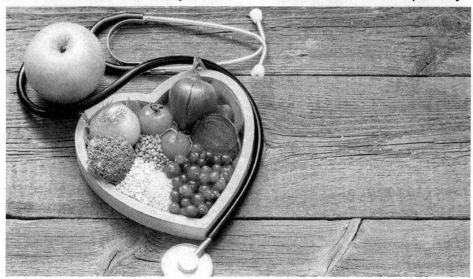

THE HEALTH BENEFITS

There are many health benefits to this diet, which include the following.

- Minimizing Hypertension: It's effective in reducing the sodium content of what you eat, which helps to control hypertension. Sodium maintains the fluid balance of your body, so high sodium equal hypertension. Less sodium naturally lowers it.

- Fighting Osteoporosis: The Dash diet is full of calcium, proteins and potassium which can fight against the onset of osteoporosis. It helps to prevent he loss of bone strength as well as form.

- Prevents Cancer: This diet is rich in antioxidants which can help to prevent cancer.

- Reduced Obesity: If you have a healthy and balanced diet, it activates the metabolism to a sharper ate which will decompose the stored fat deposits. The dash diet is rich in fibers and low on fat, so it helps you to shed the pounds, especially because exercise is still a must.

- Improved Heart: Heart conditions are often caused by the arteries, valves and veins being clogged with fat which obstructs the blood flow, and it pressurizes the heart which can cause a large list of cardiovascular disease. The Dash diet eradicates the problem by reducing your fat intake which reduces your risk of heart disease.

- Preventing Diabetes: With the Dash diet you get rid of empty carbs which decreases the amount of simple sugars that are found in your blood. This will help you to reduce your risk of diabetes.

- Helping Kidney Function: Kidneys are important to maintaining the fluid balance with the help of both sodium and potassium. When the balance is disturbed by hypertension, then the body holds onto more fluid which can cause high blood pressure. The Dash diet can improve the kidney function.

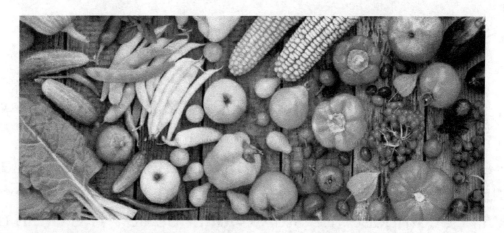

ABOUT THE PROGRAM

The Dash diet focuses on food consumption. You look at the total amount of calories and the content per meal for each serving. When you switch to the Dash diet, it's best that experts look into the routine you have, contemporary health conditions, your metabolism level, and ailments as well as exercise routines. This will help you to tailor the Dash diet to you.

WHY IT WORKS

So, you now know the basic benefits of the Dash diet, but let's take a deeper look on why the Dash diet truly works.

IT'S INCLUSIVE

There are few limitations to the diet, and there is every food item available even though some of them do have modifications. There are guides to Dos and Don'ts of this diet and ingredients. Since it's a general diet, it's inclusive to people from most walks of life.

PROMOTES EXERCISE

Like most diets that actually work, this diet does not only focus on food. It promotes physical exercise as well. With the Dash diet you get visible results because it stresses daily exercise and routine physical activities. You don't have to overdo the exercise with this diet, but daily exercise is a requirement if you want to trim the fat and help promote heart health.

PROPORTIONS

The Dash diet focuses on foods and serving sizes. Balance is key, and it's checked regularly. You must have a correct amount of all ingredients for this diet, because nothing is good in excess. Here are the servings that's been determined.

- Grains: 7-8 Daily Servings
- Fruits: 4-5 Daily Servings
- Vegetables: 4-5 Daily Servings
- Low Fat & Fat Free Dairy Products: 2-3 Daily Servings
- Meat, Poultry & Fish: 2 or Less Daily Servings
- Nuts, Seeds & Dry Beans: 4-5 Servings Per Week
- Fats & Oils: 2-3 Daily Servings
- Sweets: Less to 5 Servings per Week

Now you should look at what a serving consists of. One serving is the following.

- A slice of Bread (Not White Bread)
- 1 Cup of Fruit, Raw
- 1 cup of Vegetables, Raw
- ½ Cup Cooked Vegetables
- ½ Cup Cooked Fruit
- ½ Cup Cooked Rice
- ½ Cup Cooked Pasta
- 8 Ounces of Milk
- 3 Ounces Cooked Meat
- 3 Ounces Tofu
- 1 Teaspoon Oil

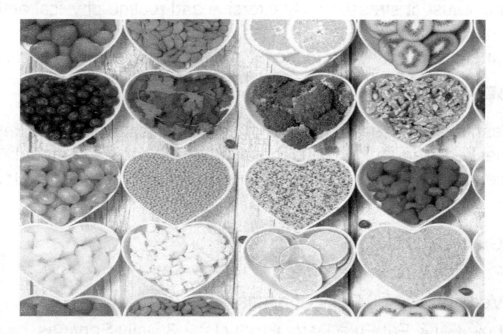

FOODS TO HAVE

Here are some foods that you should have, but remember that nothing is good in excess.

- Vegetables
- Fruits

- Poultry
- Seafood
- Seeds
- Pork
- Beef
- No Fat Dairy Products
- Low Fat Dairy Products
- Nuts
- Grains

FOODS TO AVOID

These foods you should try to limit as much as possible, and it would be better if you could cut them out of your diet all together.

- Salt
- High Fat Dairy Products
- Salted Nuts
- Sugary Beverages
- Processed Food
- Animal Based Fats (In Excess)

Dash Diet Food List-What To Avoid

21 DAY MEAL PLAN

The point of this meal plan is to help you get started with the DASH diet. If you can commit to a diet for twenty-one days, you're more than likely going to form habits that will make it easier to commit to it long term and even make it a lifestyle choice. You're allowed two snacks a day, and one of those snacks can be dessert. In this diet plan, you'll notice that snack two is before dinner, but you can move it after dinner as well. Just remember to never eat two hours before going to bed.

Versatility is also a key point in this meal plan. You'll find that many recipes used for desserts can also be a snack, many side dishes can be a snack, many lunches and dinners can be switched, and so on. There is always a little something you can add to mix up your week, even if your ingredient list is low. Of course, when looking at the dinner options, when they are just entrees, you can add sides to them to meet your requirements for the day. For example, add in a salad if you haven't had enough vegetables. Add in steamed vegetables, a cup of fruit, a little pasta, and so forth to meet your portions requirements.

DAY 1

Breakfast: Ginger Congee

Snack 1: 1 Pear

Lunch: Curry Chicken Pockets

Snack 2: Toasted Almond Ambrosia

Dinner: Beef Stir Fry

DAY 2

Breakfast: Sweet Avocado Smoothie

Snack 1: 1 Orange

Lunch: Fun Fajita Wraps

Snack 2: Apricot Biscotti

Dinner: Currant Pork Chops

DAY 3

Breakfast: Cheesy Omelet

Snack 1: 1 Apple

Lunch: Tenderloin Fajitas

Snack 2: Apple Dumplings

Dinner: Spicy Tomato Shrimp

DAY 4

Breakfast: Egg Melts

Snack 1: ½ Cup Fresh Mixed Berries

Lunch: Peanut Sauce Chicken Pasta

Snack 2: Apricot Biscotti

Dinner: Easy Barley Soup

DAY 5

Breakfast: Blueberry Muffins

Snack 1: ½ Cup Strawberries

Lunch: Vegetarian Stuffed Eggplant

Snack 2: Apple & Berry Cobbler

Dinner: Shrimp & Corn Chowder

DAY 6

Breakfast: Egg Melts

Snack 1: 1 Banana

Lunch: Vegetable Tacos

Snack 2: Squash Fries

Dinner: Coconut Shrimp

DAY 7

Breakfast: Mushroom Frittata

Snack 1: 1 Green Apple

Lunch: Chicken Cherry Wraps

Snack 2: Apple & Berry Cobbler

Dinner: Asian Salmon

DAY 8

Breakfast: Blueberry Muffins

Snack 1: 1 Asian Pear or Regular Pear

Lunch: Tuscan Stew

Snack 2: Vegetable Kebabs

Dinner: Easy Beef Brisket

DAY 9

Breakfast: Ginger Congee

Snack 1: ½ Cup Blueberry & Raspberry Mix

Lunch: Easy Barley Soup

Snack 2: Caramelized Sweet Potatoes

Dinner: Basil Halibut

DAY 10

Breakfast: Cinnamon Apple Overnight Oats

Snack 1: ½ Cup Carrot Sticks

Lunch: Arugula Risotto

Snack 2: Rosemary Potato Skins

Dinner: Beefy Fennel Stew

DAY 11

Breakfast: Pineapple Green Smoothie

Snack 1: ½ Cup Watermelon with Mint Garnish

Lunch: Fajita Style Chili

Snack 2: ½ Cup Celery Sticks with Natural Peanut Butter

Dinner: Classic Chicken Noodle Soup

DAY 12

Breakfast: Berry Quinoa Bowls

Snack 1: Vegetable Kebabs

Lunch: Vegetable Tacos

Snack 2: Pesto Mushrooms

Dinner: Asian Salmon

DAY 13

Breakfast: Yogurt & Banana Muffins

Snack 1: ½ Cup Mandarin Oranges

Lunch: Fajita Style Chili

Snack 2: ½ Cup Carrot Sticks + Sugar Free Ranch

Dinner: Coconut Shrimp

DAY 14

Breakfast: Sweet Avocado Smoothie

Snack 1: 1 Apple Sliced with All Natural Peanut Butter

Lunch: Arugula Risotto

Snack 2: Rosemary Potato Skins

Dinner: Leek & Cauliflower Soup

DAY 15

Breakfast: Yogurt & Banana Muffins

Snack 1: 1 Blood Orange or Regular Orange

Lunch: Fun Fajita Wraps

Snack 2: ½ Cup Sliced Bell Pepper

Dinner: Shrimp & Corn Chowder

DAY 16

Breakfast: Ginger Congee

Snack 1: 1 Pear Sliced & Drizzled in Honey

Lunch: Classic Chicken Noodle Soup

Snack 2: ½ Cup Honeydew Melon

Dinner: Beefy Fennel Stew

DAY 17

Breakfast: Egg Melts

Snack 1: 1 Mango

Lunch: Peanut Sauce Chicken Pasta

Snack 2: Mixed Fruit Compote Cups

Dinner: Spicy Tomato Shrimp

DAY 18

Breakfast: Berry Quinoa Bowl

Snack 1: Pesto Mushrooms

Lunch: Tuscan Stew

Snack 2: Oatmeal Surprise Cookies

Dinner: Tenderloin Fajitas

DAY 19

Breakfast: Pineapple Green Smoothie

Snack 1: Squash Fries

Lunch: Chicken Cherry Wraps

Snack 2: Blueberry Apple Cobbler

Dinner: Fennel Sauce Tenderloin

DAY 20

Breakfast: Mushroom Frittata

Snack 1: ½ Cup Sweet Peppers

Lunch: Cheesy Black Bean Wraps

Snack 2: Oatmeal Surprise Cookies

Dinner: Currant Pork Chops

DAY 21

Breakfast: Sweet Avocado Smoothie

Snack 1: ½ Cup Cantaloupe

Lunch: Tuscan Stew

Snack 2: Blueberry Apple Cobbler

Dinner: Basil Halibut

BREAKFAST RECIPES

SWEET AVOCADO SMOOTHIE

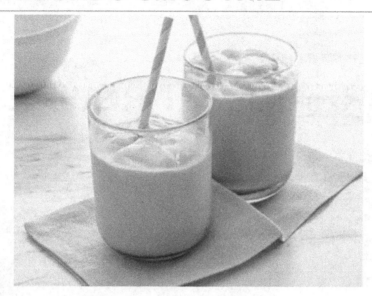

Serves: 2

Time: 5 Minutes

Calories: 323

Protein: 21 Grams

Fat: 15 Grams

Carbs: 32 Grams

Sodium: 142 mg

Cholesterol: 9 mg

Ingredients:

- 2 Cups Ice Cubes
- 1 Teaspoon Vanilla Extract, Pure
- 1 ½ Teaspoons Granulated Stevia 1 ½ Cups Milk, Nonfat
- 1 ½ Cups Peaches, Frozen
- 1 Cup Vanilla Greek Yogurt
- 1 Tablespoon Flaxseed, Ground
- 1 Avocado, Peeled & Pitted

Directions:

1. Blend all ingredients until smooth, and serve chilled.

CINNAMON APPLE OVERNIGHT OATS

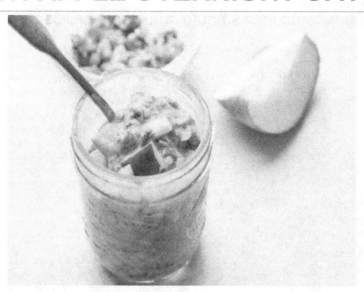

Serves: 2

Time: 8 Hours 15 Minutes

Calories: 339

Protein: 13 Grams

Fat: 8 Grams

Carbs: 60 Grams

Sodium: 66 mg

Cholesterol: 3 mg

Ingredients:

- 1 Cup Old Fashioned Rolled Oats
- 2 Tablespoons Chia Seeds
- 1 ¼ Cup Milk, Nonfat
- ½ Tablespoon Ground Cinnamon
- 2 Teaspoons Honey, Raw
- ½ Teaspoon Vanilla Extract, Pure
- Dash Sea Salt
- 1 Apple, Diced

1. Divide your chia seeds, oats, cinnamon, milk, honey, vanilla, and salt in mason jars. Place the lids on, and shake well until thoroughly combined.
2. Remove the lids, and then add half of your diced apples to each jar. Sprinkle with cinnamon. Put the lids tightly back on the jars, and refrigerate overnight.

BLUEBERRY MUFFINS

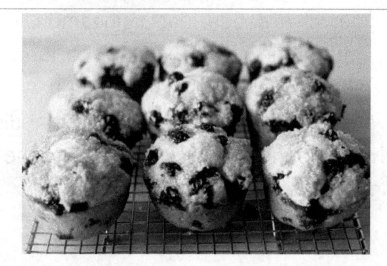

Serves: 12

Time: 45 Minutes

Calories: 180

Protein: 4 Grams

Fat: 6 Grams

Carbs: 30 Grams

Sodium: 172 mg

Cholesterol: 35 mg

Ingredients:

- 1 ¼ Cup Whole Wheat Flour
- ½ Cup Old Fashioned Rolled Oats
- 1 Teaspoon Baking Soda
- 1 Teaspoon Baking Powder
- ¼ Teaspoon Ground Cinnamon
- ¼ Teaspoon Sea Salt, Fine
- ¼ Cup Olive Oil
- ¼ Cup Dark Brown Sugar
- 1 Teaspoon Vanilla Extract, Pure

- 2 Eggs, Large
- 2/3 Cup Milk
- 1 Cup Blueberries, Fresh or Frozen
- 8 Medjool Dates, Pitted & Chopped

Directions:

1. Start by heating your oven to 350, and then line a muffin tin with liners.
2. Get out a bowl and stir your oats, flour, baking soda, baking powder, cinnamon and salt together until well combined.
3. Get out a different bowl and whisk your olive oil and brown sugar until the mixture turns fluffy. Whisk in the eggs one egg at a time until it's well beaten, and then add in your milk and vanilla extract. Beat to combine.
4. Pour your flour mixture with your wet ingredients, mixing well. Evenly spoon the batter between your muffin cups, and bake for twenty-five minutes. Allow to cool before storing.

YOGURT & BANANA MUFFINS

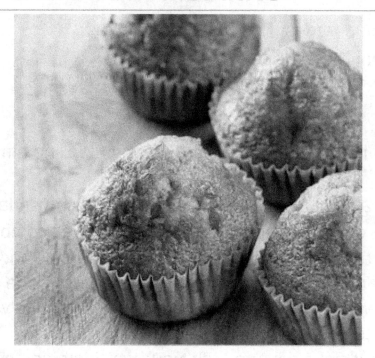

Serves: 4

Time: 40 Minutes

Calories: 316

Protein: 11.2 Grams

Fat: 14.5 Grams

Carbs: 36.8 Grams

Sodium: 469 mg

Cholesterol: 43 mg

Ingredients:

- 3 Bananas, Large & Mashed
- 1 Teaspoon Baking Soda
- 1 Cup Old Fashioned Rolled Oats
- 2 Tablespoons Flaxseed, Ground
- 1 Cup Whole Wheat Flour
- ¼ Cup Applesauce, Unsweetened

- ½ Cup Plain Yogurt
- ¼ Cup Brown Sugar
- 2 Teaspoons Vanilla Extract, Pure

Directions:

1. Start by turning the oven to 355, and then get out a muffin tray. Grease it and then get out a bowl.
2. Mix your flaxseed, oats, soda, and flour in a bowl.
3. Mash your banana and then mix in your sugar, vanilla, yogurt and applesauce. Stir in your oats mixture, making sure it's well combined. It's okay for it to be lumpy.
4. Divide between muffin trays, and then bake for twenty-five minutes. Serve warm.

BERRY QUINOA BOWLS

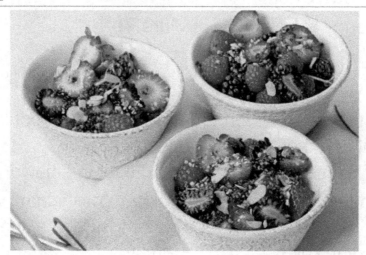

Serves: 2

Time: 35 Minutes

Calories: 435

Protein: 9.2 Grams

Fat: 13.7 Grams

Carbs: 24.9 Grams

Sodium: 141 mg

Cholesterol: 78 mg

Ingredients:

- 1 Small Peach, Sliced
- 2/3 + ¾ Cup Milk, Low Fat
- 1/3 Cup Uncooked Quinoa, Rinsed
- Well ½ Teaspoon Vanilla Extract,
- Pure 2 Teaspoons Brown Sugar
- 14 Blueberries
- 2 Teaspoons Honey, Raw
- 12 Raspberries

Directions:

1. Start to boil your quinoa, vanilla, 2/3 cup milk and brown sugar together for five minutes before reducing it to a simmer. Cook for twenty minutes.
2. Heat a grill pan that's been greased over medium heat, and then add in your peaches to grill for one minute per side.
3. Heat the remaining ¾ cup of milk in your microwave. Cook the quinoa with a splash of milk, berries and grilled peaches. Don't forget to drizzle with honey before serving it.

PINEAPPLE GREEN SMOOTHIE

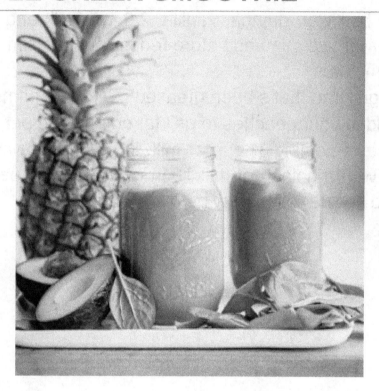

Serves: 2

Time: 5 Minutes

Calories: 213

Protein: 9 Grams

Fat: 2 Grams

Carbs: 43 Grams

Sodium: 44 mg

Cholesterol: 2.5 mg

Ingredients:

- 1 ¼ Cups Orange Juice
- ½ Cup Greek Yogurt, Plain
- 1 Cup Spinach, Fresh
- 1 Cup Pineapple, Frozen & Chunked
- 1 Cup Mango, Frozen & Chunked

- 1 Tablespoons Ground Flaxseed
- 1 Teaspoon Granulated Stevia

Directions:

1. Start by blending everything together until smooth, and then serve cold.

PEANUT BUTTER & BANANA SMOOTHIE

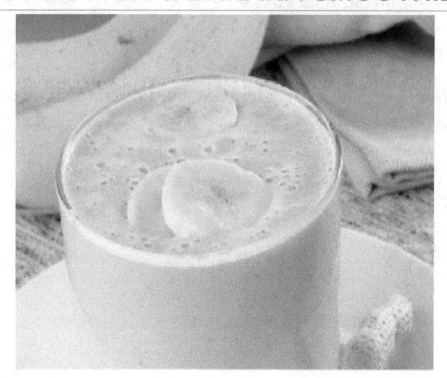

Serves: 1

Time: 5 Minutes

Calories: 146

Protein: 1.1 Grams

Fat: 5.5 Grams

Carbs: 1.8 Grams

Ingredients:

- 1 Cup Milk, Nonfat
- 1 Tablespoons Peanut Butter, All Natural
- 1 Banana, Frozen & Sliced

Directions:

1. Start by blending everything together until smooth.

MUSHROOM FRITTATA

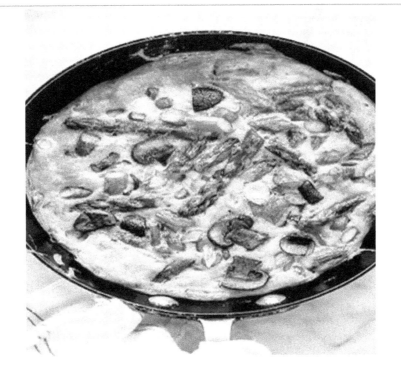

Serves: 4

Time: 30 Minutes

Calories: 391

Protein: 7.6 Grams

Fat: 12.8 Grams

Carbs: 31.5 Grams

Sodium: 32 mg

Cholesterol: 112 mg

Ingredients:

- 4 Shallots, Chopped
- 1 Tablespoons Butter
- 2 Teaspoons parsley, Fresh & Diced
- ½ lb. Mushrooms, Fresh & Diced

- 3 Eggs
- 1 Teaspoon Thyme
- 5 Egg Whites
- ¼ Teaspoon Black Pepper
- 1 Tablespoon Half & Half, Fat Free
- ¼ Cup Parmesan Cheese, Grated

Directions:

1. Start by turning the oven to 350, and then get out a skillet. Grease it with butter, letting it melt over medium heat.
2. Once your butter is hot adding in your shallots. Cook until golden brown, which should take roughly five minutes.
3. Stir in your thyme, pepper, parsley and mushrooms.
4. Beat your eggs, egg whites, parmesan, and half and half together in a bowl.
5. Pour the mixture over your mushrooms, cooking for two minutes. Transfer the skillet to the oven, and bake for fifteen minutes. Slice to serve warm.

CHEESY OMELET

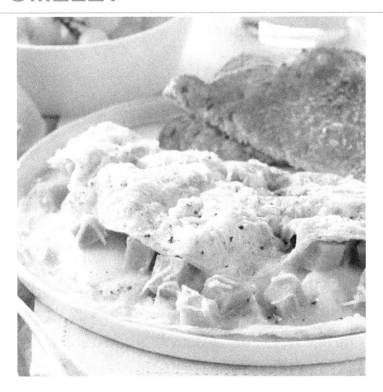

Serves: 4

Time: 20 Minutes

Calories: 427

Protein: 7.5 Grams

Fat: 8.6 Grams

Carbs: 13 Grams

Sodium: 282 mg

Cholesterol: 4.2 Grams

Ingredients:

- 4 Eggs
- 4 Cups Broccoli Florets
- 1 Tablespoons Olive Oil
- 1 Cup Egg Whites
- ¼ Cup Cheddar, Reduced Fat

- ¼ Cup Romano, Grated
- ¼ Teaspoon Sea Salt, Fine
- ¼ Teaspoon Black Pepper
- Cooking Spray as Needed

Directions:

1. Start by heating your oven to 350, and then steam your broccoli over boiling water for five to seven minutes. It should be tender.
2. Mash the broccoli into small pieces, and then toss with salt, pepper and olive oil.
3. Get out a muffin tray and then grease it with cooking spray. Divide your broccoli between the cups, and then get out a bowl.
4. In the bowl beat your eggs with salt, pepper, egg whites and parmesan.
5. Pour your batter over the broccoli, and then top with cheese. Bake for two minutes before serving warm.

GINGER CONGEE

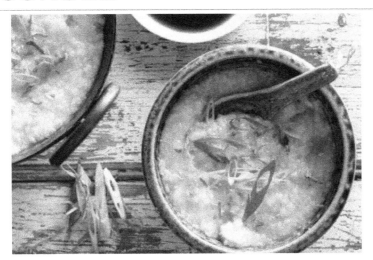

Serves: 1

Time: 1 Hour 10 Minutes

Calories: 510

protein: 13.5 Grams

Carbs: 60.7 Grams

Fat: 24.7 Grams

Sodium: 840 mg

Cholesterol: 0 mg

Ingredients:

- 1 Cup White Rice, Long Grain & Rinsed
- 7 Cups Chicken Stock
- 1 Inch Ginger, Peeled & Sliced Thin
- Green Onion, Sliced for Garnish
- Sesame Seed Oil to Garnish

Directions:

1. Start by boiling your ginger, rice and salt in a pot. Allow it to simmer and reduce to low heat. Give it a gentle stir, and then allow it to cook

for an hour. It should be thick and creamy.

2. Garnish by drizzling with sesame oil and serving warm.

EGG MELTS

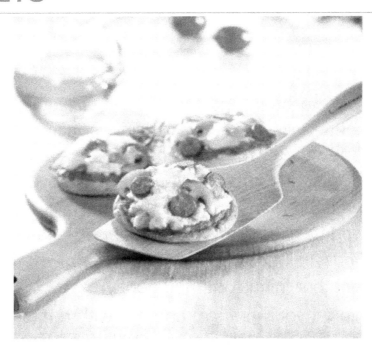

Serves: 2

Time: 20 Minutes

Calories: 212

Protein: 5.3 Grams

Fat: 3.9 Grams

Carbs: 14.3 Grams

Sodium: 135 mg

Cholesterol: 0 mg

Ingredients:

- 1 Teaspoon Olive oil
- 2 English Muffins, Whole Grain & Split
- 4 Scallions, Sliced Fine
- 8 Egg Whites, Whisked
- ¼ Teaspoon Sea Salt, Fine
- ¼ Teaspoon Black Pepper

- ½ Cup Swiss Cheese, Shredded & Reduced
- Fat ½ Cup Grape Tomatoes, Quartered

Directions:

1. Set the oven to broil, and then put your English muffins on a baking sheet. Make sure the split side is facing up. Broil for two minutes. They should turn golden around the edges.
2. Get out a skillet and grease with oil. Place it over medium heat, and cook your scallions for three minutes.
3. Beat your egg whites with salt and pepper, and pour this over your scallions.
4. Cook for another minute, stirring gently.
5. Spread this on your muffins, and top with remaining scallions if desired, cheese and tomatoes. Broil for 1 and a half more minutes to melt the cheese and serve warm.

LUNCH RECIPES

CHEESY BLACK BEAN WRAPS

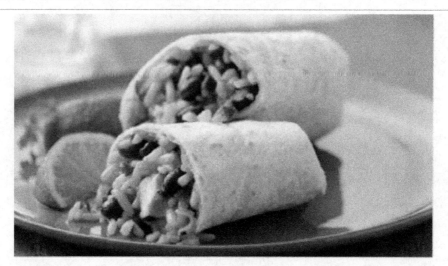

Serves: 6

Time: 15 Minutes

Calories: 341

Protein: 19 Grams

Fat: 11 Grams

Carbs: 36.5 Grams

Sodium: 141 mg

Cholesterol: 0 mg

Ingredients:

- 2 Tablespoons Green Chili Peppers, Chopped
- 4 Green Onions, Diced
- 1 Tomato, Diced
- 1 Tablespoon Garlic, Chopped
- 6 Tortilla Wraps, Whole Grain & Fat
- Free ¾ Cup Cheddar Cheese,
- Shredded ¾ Cup Salsa
- 1 ½ Cups Corn Kernels
- 3 Tablespoons Cilantro, Fresh & Chopped

- 1 ½ Cup Black Beans, Canned & Drained

Directions:

1. Toss your chili peppers, corn, black beans, garlic, tomato, onions and cilantro in a bowl.
2. Heat the mixture in a microwave for a minute, and stir for a half a minute.
3. Spread the two tortillas between paper towels and microwave for twenty seconds. Warm the remaining tortillas the same way, and add a half a cup of bean mixture, two tablespoons of salsa and two tablespoons of cheese for each tortilla. Roll them up before serving.

ARUGULA RISOTTO

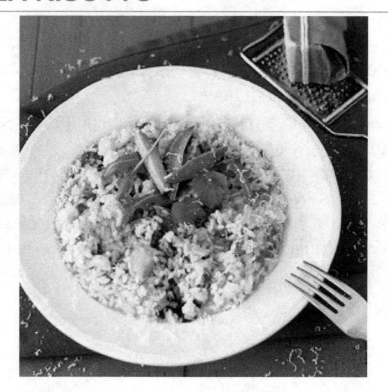

Serves: 4

Time: 25 Minutes

Calories: 288

Protein: 6 Grams

Fat: 5 Grams

Carbs: 28 Grams

Sodium: 739 mg

Cholesterol: 0.5 mg

Ingredients:

- 1 Tablespoon Olive Oil
- ½ Cup Yellow Onion, Chopped
- 1 Cup Quinoa, Rinsed
- 1 Clove Garlic, Minced
- 2 ½ Cups Vegetable Stock, Low Sodium

- 2 Cups Arugula, Chopped & Stemmed
- 1 Carrot, Peeled & shredded
- ½ Cup Shiitake Mushrooms, Sliced
- ¼ Teaspoon Black Pepper
- ¼ Teaspoon Sea Salt, Fine
- ¼ Cup Parmesan Cheese, Grated

Directions:

1. Get a saucepan and place it over medium heat, heating up your oil. Cook for four minutes until your onions are softened, and then add in your garlic and quinoa. Cook for a minute.
2. Stir in your stock, and bring it to a boil. Reduce it to simmer, and cook for twelve minutes.
3. Add in your arugula, mushrooms and carrots, cooking for an additional two minutes.
4. Add in salt, pepper and cheese before serving.

VEGETARIAN STUFFED EGGPLANT

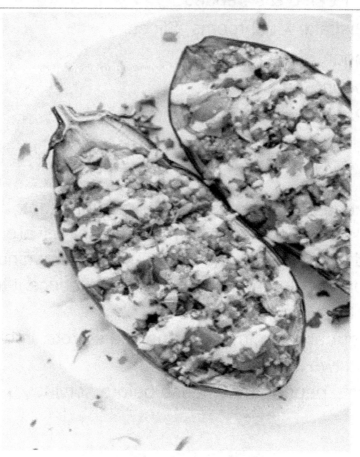

Serves: 2

Time: 35 Minutes

Calories: 334

Protein: 26 Grams

Fat: 10 Grams

Carbs: 35 Grams

Sodium: 142 mg

Cholesterol: 162 mg

Ingredients:

- 4 Ounces White Beans, Cooked
- 1 Tablespoons Olive Oil

- 1 cup Water
- 1 Eggplant
- ¼ Cup Onion, Chopped
- ½ Cup Bell Pepper, Chopped
- 1 Cup Canned Tomatoes, Unsalted
- ¼ Cup Tomato Liquid
- ¼ Cup Celery, Chopped
- 1 Cup Mushrooms, Fresh & Sliced
- ¾ Cup Breadcrumbs, Whole Wheat
- Black Pepper to Taste

Directions:

1. Preheat the oven to 350, and then grease a baking dish with cooking spray.
2. Trim the eggplant and cut it in half lengthwise. Scoop the pulp out using a spoon, leaving a shell that's a quarter of an inch thick.
3. Place the shells in the baking dish with their cut side up.
4. Add the water to the bottom of the dish, and dice the eggplant pulp into cubes, setting them to the side.
5. Add the oil into an iron skillet, heating it over medium heat.
6. Stir in peppers, chopped eggplants, and onions with your celery, mushrooms, tomatoes and tomato juice.
7. Cook for ten minutes on simmering heat, and then stir in your bread crumbs, beans and black pepper. Divide the mixture between eggshells.
8. Cover with foil, and bake for fifteen minutes. Serve warm.

VEGETABLE TACOS

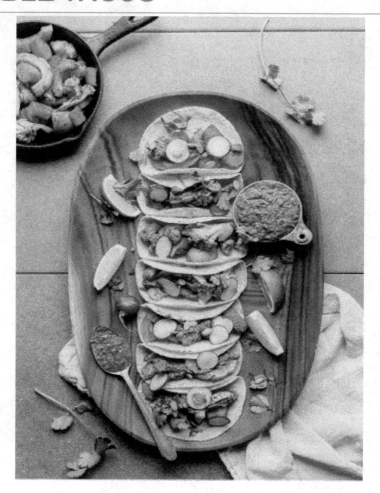

Serves: 4

Time: 30 Minutes

Calories: 310

Protein: 10 Grams

Fat: 6 Grams

Carbs: 54 Grams

Sodium: 97 mg

Cholesterol: 20 mg

Ingredients:

- 1 Tablespoon Olive Oil

- 1 Cup Red Onion, Chopped
- 1 Cup Yellow Summer Squash, Diced
- 1 Cup Green Zucchini, Diced
- 3 Cloves Garlic, Minced
- 4 Tomatoes, Seeded& Chopped
- 1 Jalapeno Chili, Seeded & Chopped
- 1 Cup Corn Kernels, Fresh
- 1 Cup Pinto Beans, Canned, Rinsed & Drained
- ½ Cup Cilantro, Fresh & Chopped
- 8 Corn Tortillas
- ½ Cup Smoke Flavored Salsa

Directions:

1. Get out a saucepan and add in your olive oil over medium heat, and stir in your onion. Cook until softened.
2. Add in your squash and zucchini, cooking for an additional five minutes.
3. Stir in your garlic, beans, tomatoes, jalapeño and corn. Cook for an additional five minutes before stirring in your cilantro and removing the pan from heat.
4. Warm each tortilla, in a nonstick skillet for twenty seconds per side.
5. Place the tortillas on a serving plate, spooning the vegetable mixture into each. Top with salsa, and roll to serve.

TUSCAN STEW

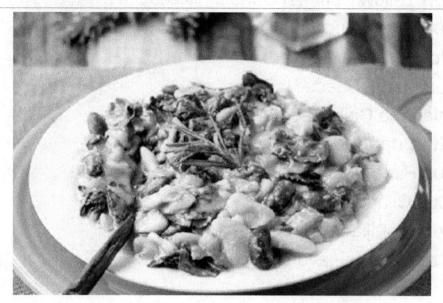

Serves: 6

Time: 1 Hour 40 Minutes

Calories: 307

Protein: 16 Grams

Fat: 7 Grams

Carbs: 45 Grams

Sodium: 463 mg

Cholesterol: 68 mg

Ingredients:

Croutons:

- 1 Tablespoons Olive Oil
- 1 Slice Bread, Whole Grain & Cubed
- 2 Cloves Garlic, Quartered

Soup:

- 1 Bay Leaf

- 2 Cups White Beans, Soaked Overnight & Drained
- 6 Cups Water
- ½ Teaspoon Sea Salt, Divided
- 1 Cup Yellow Onion, Chopped
- 2 Tablespoons Olive Oil
- 3 Carrots, Peeled & Chopped
- 6 Cloves Garlic, Chopped
- ¼ Teaspoon Ground Black Pepper
- 1 Tablespoons Rosemary, Fresh & Chopped
- 1 ½ Cups Vegetable Stock

Directions:

1. Add your oil to a skillet and heat it, and then cook your garlic for a minute. It should become fragrant. Allow it to sit for ten minutes before removing your garlic from the oil.
2. Return the pan with the oil to heat and then throw in your bread cubes. Cook for five minutes. They should be golden, and then set them to the side.
3. Mix your salt, water, bay leaf and white beans in the pot, boiling on high heat before reducing to a simmer.
4. Cover the beans and cook for one hour to one hour and ten minutes. They should be al dente.
5. Drain the beans, but reserve a half a cup of the cooking liquid. Discard the bay leaf, and transfer your beans to a bowl.
6. mix the reserved liquid with ½ cup of beans, returning it to a boil. Mash with a fork to form a paste, and then place the pot on the stove. Heat the oil using the pot.
7. Add in your onions and carrots. Cook for seven minutes and add garlic, and then cook for a minute more. Add in your rosemary, salt, pepper, stock and bean mixture.
8. Allow it to come to a boil and then reduce the heat to let it simmer. Let

it simmer for five minutes, and then top with croutons. Garnish with rosemary sprigs and enjoy.

TENDERLOIN FAJITAS

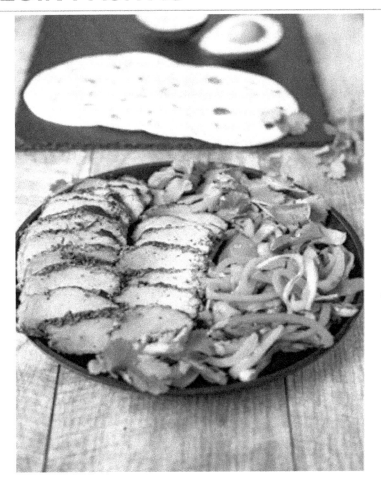

Serves: 8

Time: 35 Minutes

Calories: 250

Protein: 44 Grams

Fat: 9.8 Grams

Carbs: 21.1 Grams

Sodium: 671 mg

Cholesterol: 22 mg

Ingredients:

- ¼ Teaspoon Garlic Powder
- ¼ Teaspoon Ground Coriander

- 1 Tablespoon Chili Powder
- ½ Teaspoon Paprika
- ½ Teaspoon Oregano
- 1 lb. Pork Tenderloin, Sliced into Strips
- 8 Flour Tortillas, Whole Wheat & Warned
- 1 Small Onion, Sliced
- ½ Cup Cheddar Cheese, Shredded
- 4 Tomatoes, Diced
- 1 Cup Salsa
- 4 Cups Lettuce, Shredded

Directions:

1. Preheat a grill to 400, and then mix your coriander, garlic, oregano, paprika, and coriander in a bowl. Add in the pork slices, making sure they're well coated.
2. Arrange your pork and onions on a grilling grate, grilling for five minutes per side.
3. Stuff the tortillas with the mixture, topping with two tablespoons tomatoes, a tablespoon of cheese, ½ cup shredded lettuce and two tablespoons of salsa. Fold your tortillas and serve warm.

PEANUT SAUCE CHICKEN PASTA

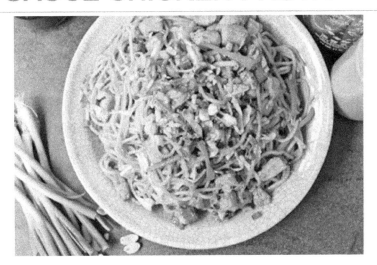

Serves: 4

Time: 30 Minutes

Calories: 403

Protein: 31 Grams

Fat: 15 Grams

Carbs: 43 Grams

Sodium: 432 mg

Cholesterol: 42 mg

Ingredients:

- 2 Teaspoons Olive Oil
- 6 Ounces Spaghetti, Whole Wheat
- 10 Ounces Snap Peas, Fresh & Trimmed & Sliced into Strips
- 2 Cups Carrots, Julienned
- 2Cups Chicken, Cooked & Shredded
- 1 Cup Thai Peanut Sauce
- 1 Cucumber, Halved Lengthwise & Sliced
- Diagonally Cilantro, Fresh & Chopped

Directions:

1. Start by cooking spaghetti as the package instructs, and then drain them and rinse the noodles using cold water.
2. Heat your greased skillet using oil, placing it over medium heat.
3. Once its hot, add in your snap peas and carrot. Cook for eight minutes, and stir in your spaghetti, chicken and peanut sauce. Toss well, and garnish with cucumber and cilantro.

CHICKEN CHERRY WRAPS

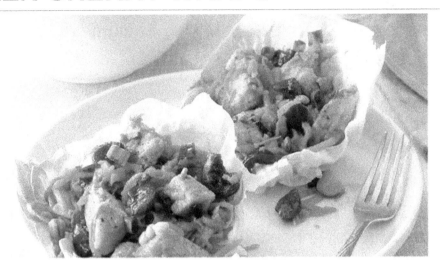

Serves: 4

Time: 20 Minutes

Calories: 257

Protein: 21 Grams

Fat: 10 Grams

Carbs: 21 Grams

Sodium: 381 mg

Cholesterol: 47 mg

Ingredients:

- ¼ Teaspoon Sea Salt, Fine
- ¼ Teaspoon Black Pepper
- 2 Teaspoons Olive oil
- ¾ lb. Chicken Breasts, Boneless &
- Cubed 1 Teaspoon Ginger, Ground 1
- ½ Cups Carrots, Shredded
- 1 ¼ Cup Sweet Cherries, Fresh, Pitted & Chopped
- 4 Green Onions, Chopped
- 2 Tablespoons Rice Vinegar

- 1/3 Cup Almonds, Chopped Roughly
- 2 Tablespoons Rice Vinegar
- 2 Tablespoons Teriyaki Sauce, Low Sodium
- 1 Tablespoon Honey Raw
- 8 Large Lettuce Leaves

Directions:

1. Season your chicken using ginger, salt and pepper.
2. Get out a skillet, placing over medium heat and adding in your oil. Once your oil is hot cook your chicken for five minutes.
3. Throw in your cherries, green onions, carrots and almonds.
4. Add in your vinegar, teriyaki and honey before making sure it's mixed well, and your chicken is cooked all the way through.
5. Spread this on lettuce leaves to serve.

EASY BARLEY SOUP

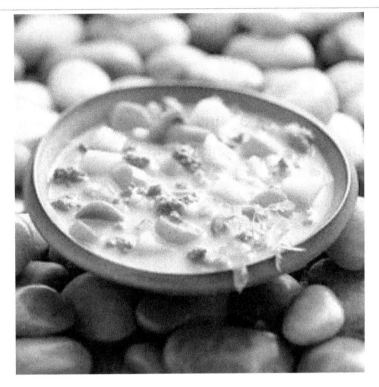

Serves: 4

Time: 30 Minutes

Calories: 208

Protein: 21 Grams

Fat: 4 Grams

Carbs: 23 Grams

Sodium: 662 mg

Cholesterol: 37 mg

Ingredients:

- 1 Tablespoon Olive Oil
- 1 Onion, Chopped
- 5 Carrots, Chopped
- 2/3 Cup Barley, Quick Cooking
- 6 Cups Chicken Broth, Reduced Sodium

- ½ Teaspoon Black Pepper
- 2 Cups Baby Spinach, Fresh
- 2 Cups Turkey Breast, Cooked & Cubed

Directions:

1. Start by getting a saucepan and heat your oil over medium high heat.
2. Stir in your carrots and onion and sauté for five minutes before adding in your barley and broth. Bring it to a boil before reducing to low to simmer. Cook for fifteen minutes.
3. Stir in your pepper, spinach and turkey. Mix well before serving.

CURRY CHICKEN POCKETS

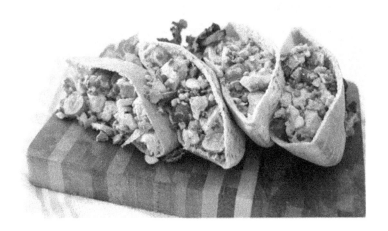

Serves: 4

Time: 35 Minutes

Calories: 415

Protein: 31.2 Grams

Fat: 32.7 Grams

Carbs: 14.7 Grams

Sodium: 277 mg

Cholesterol: 4.1 mg

Ingredients:

- 2 Cups Chicken, Cooked & Chopped
- ½ Cup Celery, Chopped
- 1/3 Cup Ricotta Cheese, Part Skim
- 1/ Cup Carrot, Shredded
- 1 Teaspoon Curry Powder
- 1 Tablespoon Apricot Preserved
- 10 Ounces Refrigerated Pizza Dough
- ¼ Teaspoon Sea Salt
- ¼ Teaspoon Ground Cinnamon

Directions:

1. Mix your carrot, ricotta, preserves, celery, chicken, cinnamon, salt and curry powder.
2. Spread the pizza dough and slice it into six equal squares.
3. Divide your mixture between each one, and then fold the corners of each towards the center and pinch them together. Put them on the baking sheet, baking at 375 for fifteen minutes. They should turn golden brown.
4. Allow them to cool before serving warm.

FAJITA STYLE CHILI

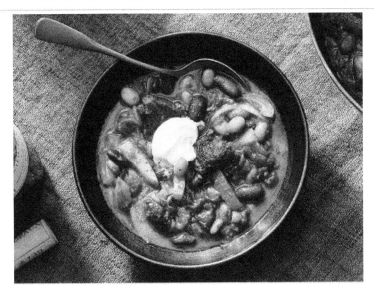

Serves: 4

Time: 5 Hours 10 Minutes

Calories: 495

Protein: 67.4 Grams

Fat: 11.5 Grams

Carbs: 10.2 Grams

Sodium: 212 mg

Cholesterol: 183 mg

Ingredients:

- 1 Teaspoon Fajita Seasoning
- 1 Tablespoon Chili Powder
- 2 lbs. Chicken Breasts, Boneless &
- Cubed ½ Teaspoon Cumin, Ground
- 2 Cloves Garlic, Minced
- Nonstick Cooking Spray as Needed
- 2 Cans (14.5 Ounces Each) Tomatoes,
- Diced ½ Green Bell Pepper, Julienned

- ½ Red Bell Pepper, Julienned
- ½ Yellow Bell Pepper, Julienned
- ½ Onion, Sliced
- 15 Ounces White Kidney Beans, Rinsed & Drained (Canned)
- 3 Tablespoons Sour Cream
- 3 Tablespoon Cheddar Cheese, Shredded & Reduced Fat
- 3 Tablespoons Guacamole

Directions:

1. mix your chicken with fajita seasoning, garlic, cumin, and chili powder.
2. Grease a skillet and place it over medium heat. Add in your chicken, cooking until it's golden brown.
3. Transfer it to a slow cooker, and then add in your tomatoes with their juices, vegetables, and beans. Cover, and cook on low for five hours.
4. Garnish with guacamole, cheese and sour cream before serving warm.

FUN FAJITA WRAPS

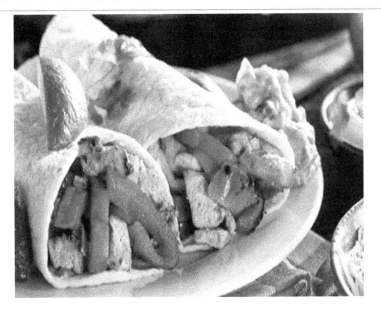

Serves: 4

Time: 20 Minutes

Calories: 245

Protein: 38.5 Grams

Fat: 16.4 Grams

Carbs: 8.7 Grams

Sodium: 471 mg

Cholesterol: 143 mg

Ingredients:

- Nonstick Cooking Spray
- ¼ Teaspoon Garlic Powder
- ½ Teaspoon Chili Powder
- 12 Ounces Chicken Breasts, Skinless & Sliced into Strips
- 1 Green Sweet Pepper, Seeded & Sliced into Strips
- 2 Tortilla, 10 Inches & Whole Wheat
- 2 Tablespoons Ranch Salad Dressing, Reduced
- Calorie ½ Cup Salsa

- 1/3 Cup Cheddar Cheese, Shredded & Reduced Fat

Directions:

1. Mix your chicken strips with chili powder and garlic powder. Heat a skillet and grease with cooking spray. Place it over medium heat, and add in your sweet pepper and chicken. Cook for six minutes.
2. Toss your salad dressing in, and divide between tortillas.
3. Top with salsa and cheese, and roll your tortilla before slicing them in half. Serve warm.

CLASSIC CHICKEN NOODLE SOUP

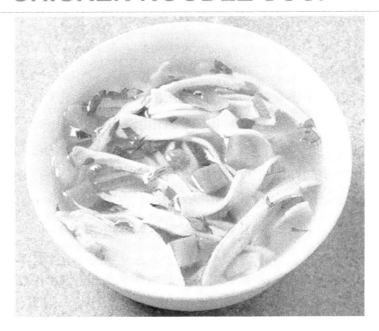

Serves: 4

Time: 30 Minutes

Calories: 381

Protein: 25.3 Grams

Fat: 12.9 Grams

Carbs: 9.7 Grams

Sodium: 480 mg

Cholesterol: 37 mg

Ingredients:

- 1 Teaspoon Olive Oil
- 1 Cup Onion, Chopped
- 3 Cloves Garlic, Minced
- 1 Cup Celery, Chopped
- 1 Cup Carrots, Sliced & Peeled
- 4 Cups Chicken Broth
- 4 Ounces Linguini, Dried & Broken

- 1 Cup Chicken Breast, Cooked & Chopped
- 2 Tablespoons Parsley, Fresh

Directions:

1. Put a saucepan over medium heat, and heat up your oil. Stir in your onion and garlic, cooking until soften.
2. Add your celery and carrots. Cook for three minutes before adding your broth. Allow it to come to a boil before reducing it to simmer. Cook for five minutes before adding in your linguini.
3. Bring it to a boil and reduce the heat to simmer. Cook for ten more minutes.
4. Add in your parsley and chicken, and then cook until heated all the way through. Serve warm.

DINNER RECIPES

FENNEL SAUCE TENDERLOIN

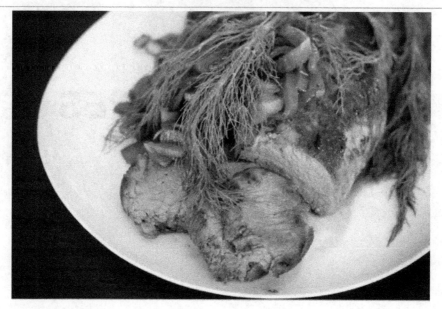

Serves: 4

Time: 35 Minutes

Calories: 276

Protein: 23.4 Grams

Fat: 24 Grams

Carbs: 14 Grams

Sodium: 647 mg

Cholesterol: 49 mg

Ingredients:

- 1 Fennel Bulb, Cored & Sliced
- 1 Sweet Onion, Sliced
- ½ Cup Dry White Wine
- 1 Teaspoon Fennel Seeds
- 4 Pork Tenderloin Fillets
- 2 Tablespoons Olive Oil
- 12 Ounces Chicken Broth, Low Sodium

- Fennel Fronds for Garnish
- Orange Slices for Garnish

Directions:

1. Thin your pork tenderloin by spreading them between parchment sheets and pounding with a mallet.
2. Heat a skillet, and add in your oil. Place it over medium heat, and cook your fennel seeds for three minutes.
3. Add the pork to the pan, cooking for an additional three minutes per side.
4. Transfer your pork to a platter before setting it to the side, and add in your fennel and onion.
5. Cook for five minutes, and then place the vegetables to the side.
6. Pour in your broth and wine, and bring it to a boil over high heat. Cook until the liquid has reduced by half.
7. Return your pork to the skillet, and cook for another five minutes.
8. Stir in your onion mixture, covering again. Cook for two more minutes, and serve warm.

BEEFY FENNEL STEW

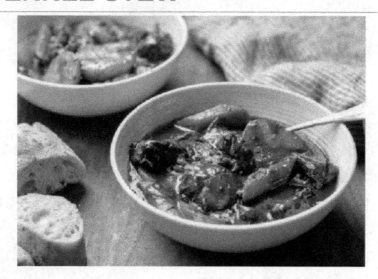

Serves: 4

Time: 1 Hour 40 Minutes

Calories: 244

Protein: 21 Grams

Fat: 8 Grams

Carbs: 22.1 Grams

Sodium: 587 mg

Cholesterol: 125 mg

Ingredients:

- 1 lb. Lean Beef, Boneless & Cubed
- 2 Tablespoons Olive Oil
- ½ Fennel Bulb, Sliced
- 3 Tablespoons All Purpose Flour
- 3 Shallots, Large & Chopped
- ¾ Teaspoon Black Pepper, Divided
- 2 Thyme Sprigs, Fresh
- 1 Bay Leaf
- ½ Cup Red Wine

- 3 Cups Vegetable Stock
- 4 Carrots, Peeled & Sliced into 1 Inch Pieces
- 4 White Potatoes, Large & Cubed
- 18 Small Boiling Onions, Halved
- 1/3 Cup Flat Leaf Parsley, Fresh & Chopped
- 3 Portobello Mushrooms, Chopped

Directions:

1. Get out a shallow container and add in your flour. Dredge the beef cubes through it, shaking off the excess flour.
2. Get out a saucepan and add in your oil, heating it over medium heat.
3. Add your beef, and cook for five minutes.
4. Add in your fennel and shallots, cooking for seven minutes. Stir in your pepper, bay leaf and thyme. Cook for a minute more.
5. Add your beef to the pan with your stock and wine.
6. Boil it and reduce it to a simmer. Cover, cooking for forty-five minutes.
7. Add in your onions, potatoes, carrots and mushrooms. Cook for another half hour, which should leave your vegetables tender.
8. Remove the thyme sprigs and bay leaf before serving warm. Carnish with parsley.

CURRANT PORK CHOPS

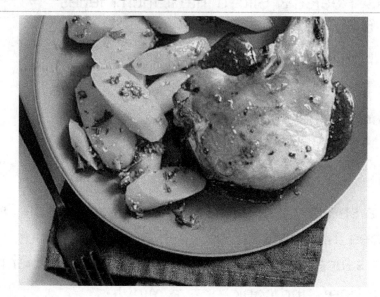

Serves: 6

Time: 30 Minutes

Calories: 265

Protein: 25 Grams

Fat: 6 Grams

Carbs: 11 Grams

Sodium: 120 mg

Cholesterol: 22 mg

Ingredients:

- 2 Tablespoons Dijon Mustard
- 6 Pork Loin Chops, Center Cut
- 2 Teaspoons Olive Oil
- 1/3 Cup Wine Vinegar
- ¼ Cup Black Currant Jam
- 6 Orange Slices
- 1/8 Teaspoon Black Pepper

Directions:

1. Start by mixing your mustard and jam together in a bowl.
2. Get out a nonstick skillet, and grease it with olive oil before placing it over medium heat. Cook your chops for five minutes per side, and then top with a tablespoon of the jam mixture. Cover, and allow it to cook for two minutes. Transfer them to a serving plate.
3. Pour your wine vinegar in the same skillet, and scape the bits up to deglaze the pan, mixing well. Drizzle this over your pork chops.
4. Garnish with pepper and orange slices before serving warm.

SPICY TOMATO SHRIMP

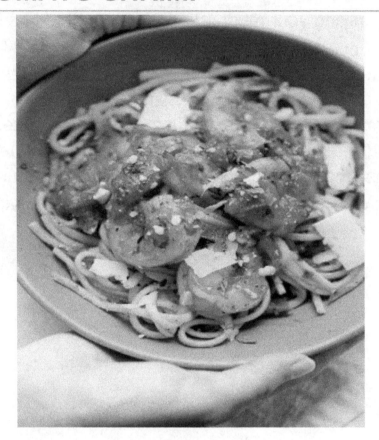

Serves: 6

Time: 35 Minutes

Calories: 185

Protein: 16.9 Grams

Fat: 1 Gram

Carbs: 12.4 Grams

Sodium: 394 mg

Cholesterol: 15 mg

Ingredients:

- ¾ lb. Shrimp, Uncooked, Peeled &
- Deveined 2 Tablespoons Tomato Paste
- ½ Teaspoon Garlic, Minced

- ½ Teaspoon Olive Oil
- 1 ½ Teaspoons Water
- ½ Teaspoon Oregano, Chopped
- ½ Teaspoon Chipotle Chili Powder

Directions:

1. Rinse and dry the shrimp before setting them to the side.
2. Get out a bowl and mix your tomato paste, water, chili powder, oil, oregano and garlic. Spread this over your shrimp, and make sure they're coated on both sides.
3. Marinate for about twenty minutes or until you're ready to grill. Preheat a gas grill to medium heat, and then grease the grate with oil. Place it six inches from the heat source. Skewer the shrimp, and for four minutes per side. Serve warm.

BEEF STIR FRY

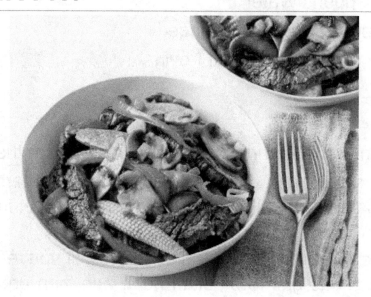

Serves: 4

Time: 40 Minutes

Calories: 408

Protein: 31 Grams

Fat: 18 Grams

Carbs: 36 Grams

Sodium: 461 mg

Cholesterol: 57 mg

Ingredients:

- 1 Head Broccoli Chopped into Florets
- 1 Red Bell Pepper, Sliced Thin
- 1 ½ Cups Brown Rice
- 2 Scallions, Sliced Thin
- 2 Tablespoons Sesame Seeds
- ¼ Teaspoon Black Pepper
- 1 lb. Flank Steak, Sliced Thin
- 2 Tablespoons Canola Oil

- ¾ Cup Stir Fry Sauce

Directions:

1. Start by heating your oil in a large wok over medium-high heat. Add in your steak, seasoning with pepper. Cook for four minutes or until crisp. Remove it from the skillet.
2. Place your broccoli in the skillet and cook for four minutes. Toss occasionally. It should be tender but crisp.
3. Put your steak back in the skillet, and pour in your sauce. Allow it to simmer for three minutes.
4. Serve over rice with sesame seeds and scallions.

SHRIMP & CORN CHOWDER

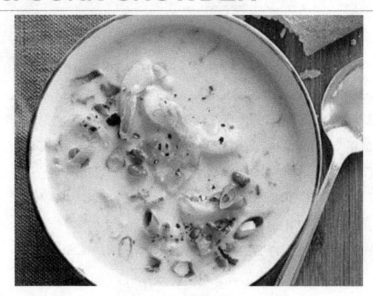

Serves: 6

Time: 50 Minutes

Calories: 340

Protein: 23 Grams

Fat: 9 Grams

Carbs: 45 Grams

Sodium: 473 mg

Cholesterol: 115 mg

Ingredients:

- 2 Carrots, Peeled & Sliced
- 1 Yellow Onion, Sliced
- 3 Tablespoons Olive Oil
- 2 Celery Stalks, Diced
- 4 Baby Red Potatoes, Diced
- 4 Cloves Garlic, Peeled & Minced
- ¼ Cup All Purpose Flour
- 3 Cups Vegetable Stock, Unsalted

- ½ Cup Milk
- ¾ Teaspoon Sea Salt, Fine
- ¼ Teaspoon Black Pepper
- ¼ Teaspoon Cayenne Pepper
- 4 Cups Corn Kernels Fresh
- 1 lb. Shrimp, Peeled & Deveined
- 2 Scallions Sliced Thin

Directions:

1. Get out a stockpot and heat your oil using medium heat. Once your oil is hot adding in your carrots, celery, potatoes and onion. Cook for seven minutes. The vegetable should soften. Stir and then add in your garlic. Cook for a minute more.
2. Make a flour roux, and increase the heat to medium high. Whisk and bring it to a simmer. Make sure to whisk any lumps out. Whisk in your milk, salt, pepper and cayenne. Allow it to simmer until it thickens. This should take about eight minutes.
3. Add in your shrimp and corn, and cook for another five minutes.
4. Divide between bowls to serve warm.

LEEK & CAULIFLOWER SOUP

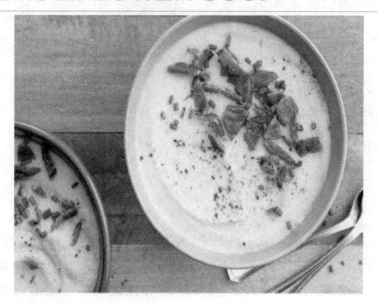

Serves: 6

Time: 40 Minutes

Calories: 92

Protein: 5 Grams

Fat: 4 Grams

Carbs: 13 Grams

Sodium: 556 mg

Cholesterol: 3 mg

Ingredients:

- 1 Tablespoon Olive Oil
- 1 Leek, Trimmed & Sliced Thin
- 1 Yellow Onion, Peeled & Diced
- 1 Head Cauliflower, Chopped into Florets
- 3 Cloves Garlic, Minced
- 2 Tablespoons Thyme, Fresh & Chopped
- 1 Teaspoon Smoked Paprika
- 1 ¼ Teaspoons Sea Salt, Fine

- 1/4 Teaspoon Ground Cayenne Pepper
- 1 Tablespoon Heavy Cream
- 3 Cups Vegetable Stock, Unsalted
- ½ Lemon, Juiced & Zested

Directions:

1. Heat your oil in a stockpot over medium heat, and add in your leek, onion, and cauliflower. Cook for five minutes or until the onion begins to soften. Add in your garlic, thyme, smoked paprika, salt, pepper and cayenne. Pour in your vegetable stock and bring it to a simmer, cooking for fifteen minutes. Your cauliflower should be very tender.
2. Remove from heat and stir in your lemon juice, lemon zest and cream. Use an immersion blender to puree, and serve warm.

EASY BEEF BRISKET

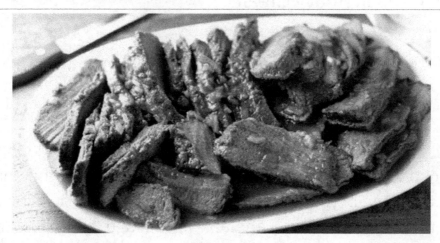

Serves: 4

Time: 3 Hours 10 Minutes

Calories: 299

Protein: 10.2 Grams

Fat: 9 Grams

Carbs: 21.4 Grams

Sodium: 372 mg

Cholesterol: 101 mg

Ingredients:

- 1 Teaspoon Thyme
- 4 Cloves Garlic, Peeled & Smashed
- 1 ½ Cups Onion, chopped
- 2 ½ lbs. Beef Brisket, Chopped
- 1 Tablespoons Olive Oil
- ¼ Teaspoon Black Pepper
- 14.5 Ounces Tomatoes & Liquid,
- Canned ¼ Cup Red Wine Vinegar
- 1 Cup Beef Stock, Low Sodium

Directions:

1. Turn the oven to 350, and then grease a Dutch oven using a tablespoon of oil. Place it over medium heat.
2. Add in your pepper and brisket. Cook until it browns, and then place your brisket on a plate.
3. Put your onions in the pot, and cook until golden brown. Stir in your garlic and thyme, cooking for another full minute before adding in the stock, vinegar and tomatoes.
4. Cook until it comes to a boil and add in your brisket again.
5. Reduce to a simmer, and cook for three hours in the oven until tender.

COCONUT SHRIMP

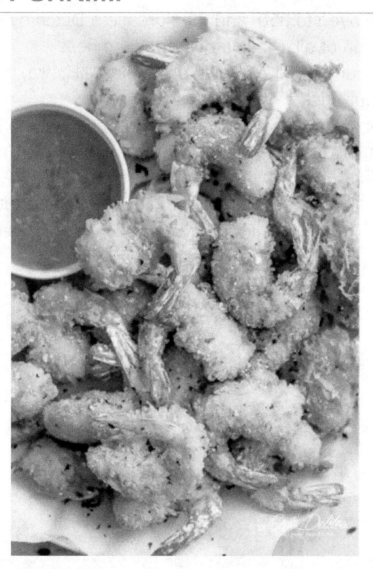

Serves: 4

Time: 25 Minutes

Calories: 249

Protein: 35 Grams

Fat: 1.7 Grams

Carbs: 1.8 Grams

Sodium: 79 mg

Cholesterol: 78 mg

Ingredients:

- ¼ Cup Coconut, Sweetened
- ½ Teaspoon Sea Salt, Fine
- ¼ Cup Panko Breadcrumbs
- ½ Cup Coconut Milk
- 12 Large Shrimp, Peeled & Deveined

Directions:

1. Preheat your oven to 375, and then get out a baking pan. Spray it with cooking spray before setting it aside.
2. Grind your panko with coconut and salt in a food processor.
3. Add this mixture to a bowl and pour the coconut milk in another bowl.
4. Dip the shrimp in the coconut mixture and then dredge it through the panko mixture. Put the coated shrimp on the baking pan, and then bake for fifteen minutes. Serve warm.

ASIAN SALMON

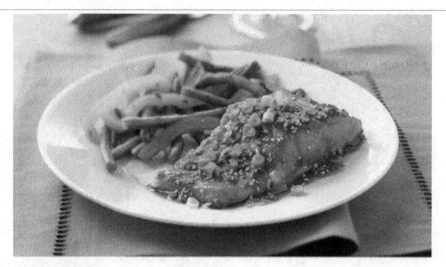

Serves: 2

Time: 30 Minutes

Calories: 247

Protein: 27 Grams

Fat: 7 Grams

Carbs: 19 Grams

Sodium: 350 mg

Cholesterol: 120 mg

Ingredients:

- 1 Cup Fresh Fruit, Diced
- ¼ Teaspoon Black Pepper
- 2 Salmon Fillets, 4 Ounces Each
- ¼ Teaspoon Sesame Oil
- 1 Teaspoon Soy Sauce, Low Sodium
- 2 Cloves Garlic, Minced
- ½ Cup Pineapple Juice, Sugar Free

Directions:

1. Start by getting out a bowl and mix your garlic, soy sauce, ginger and pineapple juice together. Place your fish in the doughs and make sure it's covered. It marinates for an hour.
2. Flip the fillets after thirty minutes, and then heat the oven to 375.
3. Get out aluminum squares and grease them with cooking spray. Put the salmon fillet on each square, and drizzle with pepper, diced fruit and sesame oil. Fold the aluminum sheet to seal the fish, and then place them on the baking sheet.
4. Bake for ten minutes per side before serving.

BASIL HALIBUT

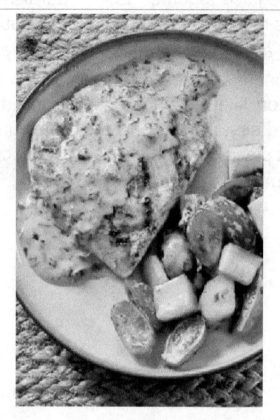

Serves: 4

Time: 30 Minutes

Calories: 128

Protein: 21 Grams

Fat: 4 Grams

Carbs: 3 Grams

Sodium: 81 mg

Cholesterol: 55 mg

Ingredients:

- 4 Halibut Fillets, 4 Ounces Each
- 2 Teaspoons Olive Oil
- 1 Tablespoon Garlic, Minced
- 2 Tomatoes, Diced

- 2 Tablespoons Basil, Fresh & Chopped
- 1 Teaspoon Oregano, Fresh & Chopped

Directions:

1. Heat the oven to 350, and then get out a 9 by 13-inch pan. Spray it down with cooking spray.
2. Toss the basil, olive oil garlic, oregano and tomato together in a bowl. Pour this over your fish in the pan.
3. Bake the twelve minutes. Your fish should be flakey.

SIDE DISH RECIPES

PESTO MUSHROOMS

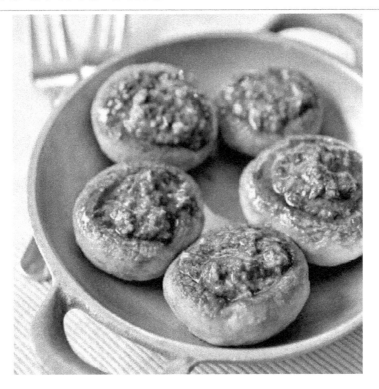

Serves: 10

Time: 25 Minutes

Calories: 159

Protein: 2 Grams

Fat: 3 Grams

Carbs: 4 Grams

Sodium: 63 mg

Cholesterol: 8 mg

Ingredients:

20 Cremini Mushrooms, Washed & Stemmed

Toppings:

- 1 ½ Cups Panko Breadcrumbs
- ¼ Cup Butter, Melted

- 3 Tablespoons Parsley, Fresh & Chopped

Filling:

- 2 Cups Basil Leaves, Fresh & Chopped
- ¼ Cup Parmesan Cheese, Grated Fresh
- 2 Tablespoons Pumpkin Seeds
- 1 Tablespoon Garlic, Fresh
- 1 Tablespoon Olive Oil
- 2 Teaspoons Lemon Juice, Fresh
- ½ Teaspoon Sea Salt, Fine

Directions:

1. Turn your oven to3 50, and then arrange your mushrooms on a baking sheet with the caps up.
2. Prepare the topping by getting out a bowl and mixing your parsley, panko and butter.
3. Mix your pumpkin seeds, cheese, garlic, oil, basil, lemon juice and slat in a blender, blending until well combined.
4. Stuff the mushrooms with the basil paste before topping with the panko mixture.
5. Press this into the caps, and bake for fifteen minutes. They should turn golden brown before serving warm.

LEMON GREEN BEANS WITH ALMONDS

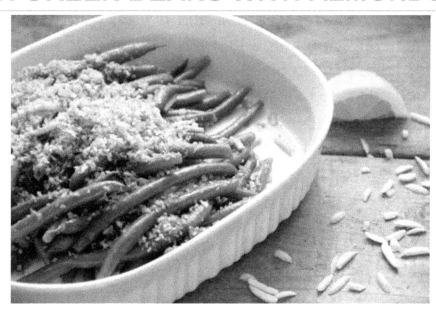

Serves: 4

Time: 30 Minutes

Calories: 162

Protein: 6 Grams

Fat: 11 Grams

Carbs: 10 Grams

Sodium: 132 mg

Cholesterol: 0 mg

Ingredients:

- ¼ Cup Parmesan Cheese, Grated Fine
- ¼ Cup Almonds, Sliced
- ¼ Teaspoon Black Pepper
- 1/8 Teaspoon Sea Salt, Fine
- 1 Lemon, Juiced & Zested
- 2 Tablespoons Olive Oil
- 1 lb. Green Beans, Trimmed

Directions:

1. Bring a pot of water to a boil and blanch your green beans for three minutes. Submerge them in a bowl of ice water for three minutes to stop the cooking and drain.
2. Heat your olive oil in a skillet using medium heat. Add in your green beans and sauté for five minutes or until browned lightly.
3. Add in your lemon juice, and allow it to cook for two more minutes. Season with salt and pepper.
4. Transfer it to a serving dish and top with lemon zest, parmesan, and almonds.

SWEET & SAVORY BRUSSEL SPROUTS

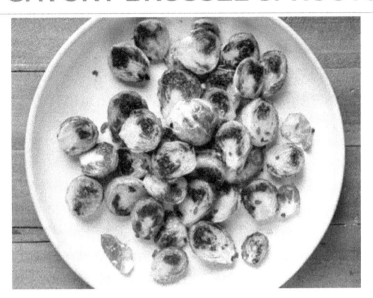

Serves: 6

Time: 30 Minutes

Calories: 151

Protein: 6 Grams

Fat: 8 Grams

Carbs: 16 Grams

Sodium: 255 mg

Cholesterol: 0 mg

Ingredients:

- ¼ Cup Walnuts, Chopped
- 2 Tablespoons Olive Oil
- 2 lbs. Brussel Sprouts, Trimmed &
- Halved ¼ Teaspoon Black Pepper ¼
- Teaspoon Sea Salt, Fine
- 1/8 Teaspoon Crushed Red Pepper Flakes
- 1 Tablespoon Maple Syrup, Pure
- 2 Tablespoons Dijon Mustard

Directions:

1. Heat a dry skillet over medium heat, and then toast your walnuts for two minutes. They should be lightly toasted, and then place them in a small bowl.
2. Heat your olive oil over a skillet over medium heat, and add in the Brussel sprouts. Cook for ten minutes, and stir occasionally. They should be browned and fork tender. Season with salt, pepper and red pepper.
3. Get out a bowl and whisk your Dijon mustard and maple syrup, and then pour in the pan. Stir until well combined, and bring to a light simmer.
4. Transfer this to a dish and top with your toasted walnuts.

CARAMELIZED SWEET POTATOES

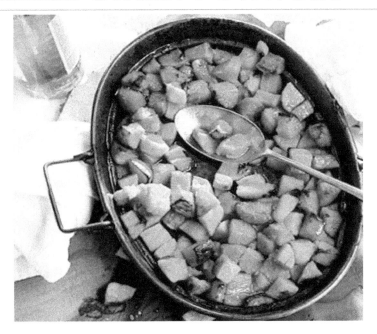

Serves: 4

Time: 55 Minutes

Calories: 111

Protein: 1 Grams

Fat: 7 Grams

Carbs: 12 Grams

Sodium: 166 mg

Cholesterol: 0 mg

Ingredients:

- 2 Sweet potatoes, Cut into ½ Inch
- Wedges 2 Tablespoons Canola Oil ¼
- Teaspoon Black Pepper ¼ Teaspoon
- Sea Salt, Fine

Directions:

1. Preheat your oven to 450, and then line a baking sheet with a with a

wire rack. Spray your wire wrack down with cooking spray.

2. Coat your sweet potatoes in oil before seasoning with salt and pepper, and then place them an inch apart on the rack. Bake for thirty to thirty-five minutes.

3. Turn the oven to a low broil, cooking for four minutes more. The edges should be browned. Serve warm.

VEGETABLE & POLENTA DISH

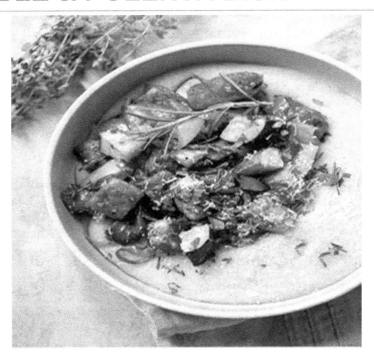

Serves: 4

Time: 1 Hour

Calories: 178

Protein: 6 Grams

Fat: 1 Gram

Carbs: 22 Grams

Sodium: 326 mg

Cholesterol: 14 mg

Ingredients:

- 2 Tablespoons Parmesan Cheese, Grated
- 1 Cup Zucchini, Sliced
- 1 Cup Broccoli Florets, Chopped
- 1 Cup Onions, Sliced
- 1 Cup Mushrooms, Fresh & Sliced
- ½ Teaspoon Oregano, Fresh & Chopped

- 1 Teaspoon Basil, Fresh & Chopped
- ½ Teaspoon Rosemary, Fresh & Chopped
- 1 Cup Polenta, Ground Coarsely
- 4 Cups water
- 1 Teaspoon Garlic, Chopped

Directions:

1. Heat the oven to 350, and then grease a three-quart baking dish with cooking spray. Mix the polenta, garlic and water. Bake for forty minutes, and then heat a skillet that's been greased over medium heat.
2. Add in your mushrooms and onions, cooking for five minutes.
3. Boil the water in a pot and then add in the steamer basket.
4. Put your zucchini and broccoli in the basket, steaming for three minutes while covered.
5. Bake your polenta with the steamed vegetable, and garnish with cheese and herbs. Serve warm.

ROSEMARY POTATO SKINS

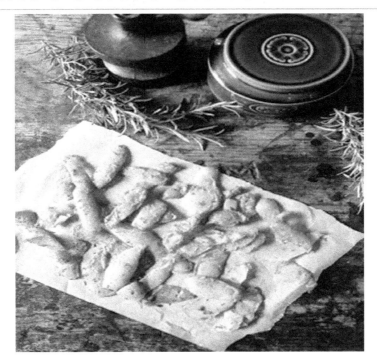

Serves: 2

Time: 1 Hour 10 Minutes

Calories: 167

Protein: 7.6 Grams

Fat: 0 Grams

Carbs: 27 Grams

Sodium: 119 mg

Cholesterol: 20 mg

Ingredients:

- 2 Russet Potatoes
- Butter Flavored Cooking Spray
- 1 Tablespoon Rosemary, Fresh &
- Minced 1/8 Teaspoon Black Pepper

Directions:

1. Heat your oven to 375, and then pierce your potatoes with a fork. Place them on a baking sheet and bake for an hour until crispy.
2. Allow them to cool and then cut them in half lengthwise.
3. Scoop the pulp out and leave 1/8 inch of a shell.
4. Brush the shells with melted butter and season with rosemary and pepper. Reserve the flesh for another recipe or time.
5. Bake for another five minutes before serving.

SQUASH FRIES

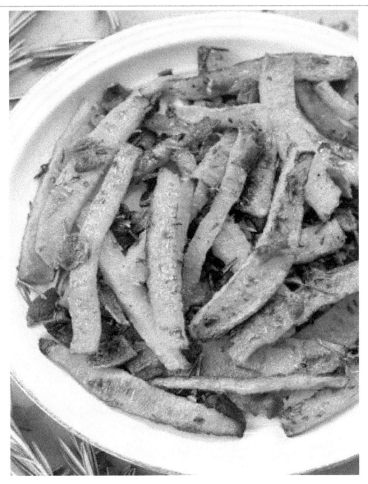

Serves: 4

Time: 25 Minutes

Calories: 62

Protein: 11 Grams

Fat: 2 Grams

Carbs: 11 Grams

Sodium: 38 mg

Cholesterol: 1 mg

Ingredients:

- 1 Tablespoons Rosemary, Fresh & Chopped

- 1 Tablespoon Thyme, Fresh & Chopped
- 1 Tablespoon Olive Oil
- 1 Butternut Squash
- ½ Teaspoon Sea Salt, Fine

Directions:

1. Turn the oven to 425 degrees, and then get out a baking sheet. Grease it.
2. Peel your squash and slice it into ½ inch wide and three inch long pieces.
3. Put the pieces in a bowl and toss with salt, thyme, oil and rosemary.
4. Spread your squash on the baking sheet, baking for ten minutes.
5. Toss, and bake for five minutes more. They should be golden brown.

VEGETABLE KEBABS

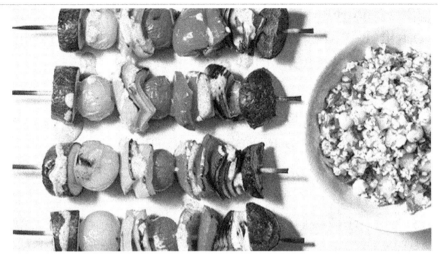

Serves: 2

Time: 55 Minutes

Calories: 335

Protein: 8.8 Grams

Fat: 8.2 Grams

Carbs: 67 Grams

Sodium: 516 mg

Cholesterol: 110 mg

Ingredients:

- 1 Zucchini, Sliced into pieces
- 1 Red Onion, Quartered
- 1 Green bell Pepper, Cut into 4 Pieces
- 8 Button Mushrooms
- 8 Cherry Tomatoes
- ½ Cup Italian Dressing, Fat Free
- 1 Red Bell Pepper, Cut into 4 Pieces
- ½ Cup Brown Rice
- 1 Cup Water

Directions:

1. Toss the zucchini, mushrooms, onion, peppers, and tomatoes with your Italian dressing in a bowl, allowing them to marinate for ten minutes. Make sure they're well coated.
2. Boil the water with rice in a saucepan, reducing it to simmer. Cook covered for a half hour or until your rice is done.
3. Prepare your grill by preheating it to medium.
4. Grease the grilling rack with cooking spray and position it four inches from heat.
5. Thread two tomatoes, two mushrooms, two zucchini slices, 1 onion wedge, one green pepper and one red pepper slice per skewer. Grill for five minutes per side.
6. Serve with rice while warm.

DESSERT RECIPES

TOASTED ALMOND AMBROSIA

Serves: 2

Time: 30 Minutes

Calories: 177

Protein: 3.4 Grams

Fat: 4.9 Grams

Carbs: 36 Grams

Sodium: 13 mg

Cholesterol: 11 mg

Ingredients:

- ½ Cup Almonds, Slivered
- ½ Cup Coconut, Shredded & Unsweetened
- 3 Cups Pineapple, Cubed
- 5 Oranges, Segment
- 1 Banana, Halved Lengthwise, Peeled & Sliced
- 2 Red Apples, Cored & Diced
- 2 Tablespoons Cream Sherry
- Mint Leaves, Fresh to Garnish

Directions:

1. Start by heating your oven to 325, and then get out a baking sheet. Roast your almonds for ten minutes, making sure they're spread out evenly.
2. Transfer them to a plate and then toast your coconut on the same baking sheet. Toast for ten minutes.
3. Mix your banana, sherry, oranges, apples and pineapple in a bowl.
4. Divide the mixture not serving bowls and top with coconut and almonds.

5. Garnish with mint before serving.

APPLE DUMPLINGS

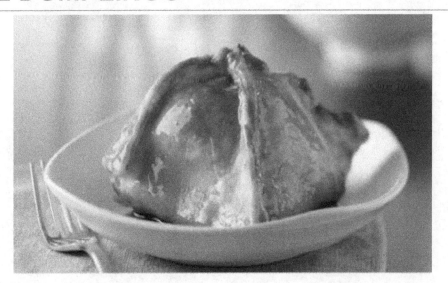

Serves: 4

Time: 40 Minutes

Calories: 178

Protein: 5 Grams

Fat: 4 Grams

Carbs: 23 Grams

Sodium: 562 mg

Cholesterol: 61 mg

Ingredients:

Dough:

- 1 Tablespoon Butter
- 1 Teaspoon Honey, Raw
- 1 Cup Whole Wheat Flour
- 2 Tablespoons Buckwheat Flour
- 2 Tablespoons Rolled Oats
- 2 Tablespoons Brandy or Apple Liquor

Filling:

- 2 Tablespoons Honey, Raw
- 1 Teaspoon Nutmeg
- 6 Tart Apples, Sliced Thin
- 1 Lemon, Zested

Directions:

1. Turn the oven to 350.
2. Get out a food processor and mix your butter, flours, honey and oats until it forms a crumbly mixture.
3. Add in your brandy or apple liquor, pulsing until it forms a dough.
4. Seal in a plastic and place it in the fridge for two hours.
5. Toss your apples in lemon zest, honey and nutmeg.
6. Roll your dough into a sheet that's a quarter inch thick. Cut out eight-inch circles, placing each circle into a muffin tray that's been greased.
7. Press the dough down and then stuff with the apple mixture. Fold the edges, and pinch them closed. Make sure that they're well sealed.
8. Bake for a half hour until golden brown, and serve drizzled in honey.

APRICOT BISCOTTI

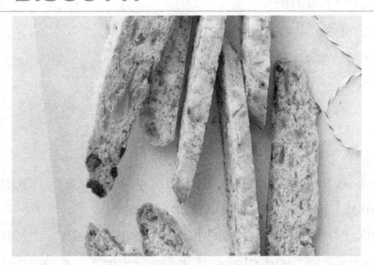

Serves: 4

Time: 50 Minutes

Calories: 291

Protein: 2 Grams

Fat: 2 Grams

Carbs: 12 Grams

Sodium: 123 mg

Cholesterol: 21 mg

Ingredients:

- 2 Tablespoons Honey, Dark
- 2 Tablespoons Olive Oil
- ½ Teaspoon Almond Extract
- ¼ Cup Almonds, Chopped Roughly
- 2/3 Cup Apricots, Dried
- 2 Tablespoons Milk, 1% & Low Fat
- 2 Eggs, Beaten Lightly
- ¾ Cup Whole Wheat Flour
- ¾ Cup All Purpose Flour

- ¼ Cup Brown Sugar, Packed Firm
- 1 Teaspoon Baking Powder

Directions:

1. Start by heating the oven to 350, and then mix your baking powder, brown sugar and flours in a bowl.
2. Whisk your canola oil, eggs, almond extract, honey and milk. Mix well until it forms a smooth dough. Fold in the apricots and almonds.
3. Put your dough on plastic wrap, and then roll it out to a twelve inch long and three inch wide rectangle. Place this dough on a baking sheet, and bake for twenty-five minutes. It should turn golden brown. Allow it to cool, and slice it to ½ inch thick slices, and then bake for another fifteen minutes. It should be crispy.

APPLE & BERRY COBBLER

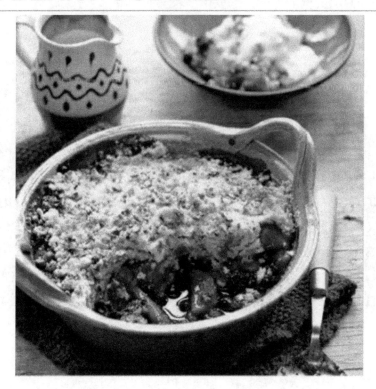

Serves: 4

Time: 40 Minutes

Calories: 131

Protein: 7.2 Grams

Fat: 1 Grams

Carbs: 13.8 Grams

Sodium: 14 mg

Cholesterol: 2.1 mg

Ingredients:

Filling:

- 1 Cup Blueberries, Fresh
- 2 Cups Apples, Chopped
- 1 Cup Raspberries, Fresh
- 2 Tablespoons Brown Sugar

- 1 Teaspoon Lemon Zest
- 2 Teaspoon Lemon Juice, Fresh
- ½ Teaspoon Ground Cinnamon
- 1 ½ Tablespoons Corn Starch

Topping:

- ¾ Cup Whole Wheat Pastry Flour
- 1 ½ Tablespoons Brown Sugar
- ½ Teaspoon Vanilla Extract, Pure
- ¼ Cup Soy Milk
- ¼ Teaspoon Sea Salt, Fine
- 1 Egg White

Directions:

1. Turn your oven to 350, and get out six small ramekins. Grease them with cooking spray.
2. Mix your lemon juice, lemon zest, blueberries, sugar, cinnamon, raspberries and apples together in a bowl.
3. Stir in your cornstarch, mixing until it dissolves.
4. Beat your egg white in a different bowl, whisking it with sugar, vanilla, soy milk and pastry flour.
5. Divide your berry mixture between the ramekins and top with the vanilla topping.
6. Put your ramekins on a baking sheet, baking for thirty minutes. The top should be golden brown before serving.

MIXED FRUIT COMPOTE CUPS

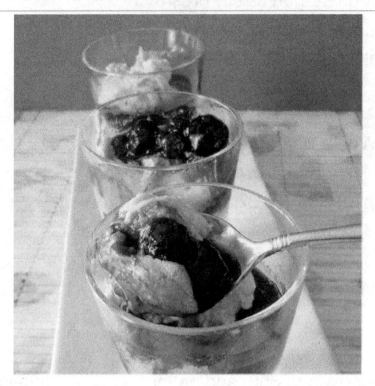

Serves: 2

Time: 15 Minutes

Calories: 228

Protein: 9.1 Grams

Fat: 5.7 Grams

Carbs: 12.4 Grams

Sodium: 114 mg

Cholesterol: 15 mg

Ingredients:

- 1 ¼ Cup Water
- ½ Cup Orange juice
- 12 Ounces Mixed Dried Fruit
- 1 Teaspoon Ground Cinnamon
- ¼ Teaspoon Ground Ginger

- ¼ Teaspoon Ground Nutmeg
- 4 Cups Vanilla Frozen Yogurt, Fat Free

Directions:

1. Mix your dried fruit, nutmeg, cinnamon, water, orange juice and ginger in a saucepan.
2. Cover, and allow it to cook over medium heat for ten minutes. Remove the cover, and then cook for another ten minutes.
3. Add your frozen yogurt to serving cups, and top with the fruit mixture.

OATMEAL SURPRISE COOKIES

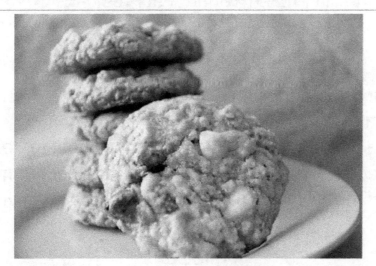

Serves: 24

Time: 25 Minutes

Calories: 152

Protein: 4 Grams

Fat: 10 Grams

Carbs: 12 Grams

Sodium: 131 mg

Cholesterol: 18 mg

Ingredients:

- 1 ½ Cups Creamy Peanut Butter, All
- Natural ½ Cup Dark Brown Sugar
- 2 Eggs, Large
- 1 Cup Old Fashioned Rolled Oats
- 1 Teaspoon Baking Soda
- ½ Teaspoon Sea Salt, Fine
- ½ Cup Dark Chocolate Chips

Directions:

1. Start by heating your oven to 350, and get out a baking sheet. Line your baking sheet with parchment paper.
2. Get out a bowl with an electric mixer and whip your peanut butter until smooth. Continue beating as you add in your brown sugar. Keep beating as you add in one egg at a time until it's incorporated and fluffy. Beat in your oats, salt and baking soda. Turn the mixer off and fold in your dark chocolate chips.
3. Put your cookie dough on a baking sheet two inches apart and bake for eight to ten minutes.

ALMOND & APRICOT CRISP

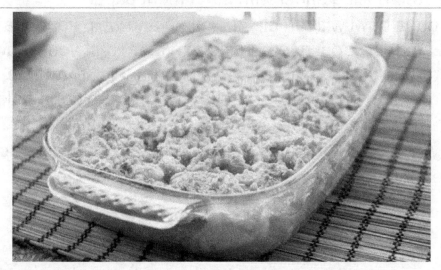

Serves: 4

Time: 35 Minutes

Calories: 149

Protein: 3 Grams

Fat: 11.9 Grams

Carbs: 18.8 Grams

Sodium: 79 mg

Cholesterol: 78 mg

Ingredients:

- 1 Teaspoon Olive Oil
- 1 lb. Apricot, Halved & Pits Removed
- ½ Cup Almonds, Chopped
- 1 Tablespoons Oats
- 1 Teaspoon Anise Seeds
- 2 Tablespoons Honey, Raw

Directions:

1. start by heating the oven to 350, and then grease a nine-inch pie plate

with olive oil.

2. Add in your apricots once they're chopped, and spread them out evenly.

3. Top with anise seeds, oats and almonds. Pour honey on top, and bake for twenty-five minutes. It should turn golden brown.

BLUEBERRY APPLE COBBLER

Serves: 4

Time: 40 Minutes

Calories: 288

Protein: 6 Grams

Fat: 6.2 Grams

Carbs: 48 Grams

Sodium: 176 mg

Cholesterol: 120 mg

Ingredients:

- 2 Tablespoons Cornstarch
- 2 Tablespoons Sugar
- 1 Tablespoon Lemon Juice, Fresh
- 2 Apples, Large, Peeled, Cored & Sliced
- 1 Teaspoon Ground Cinnamon
- 12 Ounces Blueberries, Fresh

Toppings:

- ¼ Teaspoon Sea Salt, Fine
- ¾ Cup All Purpose Flour
- ¾ Cup Whole Wheat Flour
- 2 Tablespoons Sugar
- 1 ½ Teaspoons Baking Powder
- 4 Tablespoons Margarine, Cold &
- Chopped ½ Cup Milk, Fat Free
- 1 Teaspoon Vanilla Extract, Pure

Directions:

1. Turn the oven to 400 degrees, and then get out a nine-inch baking pan. Grease it using cooking spray.
2. Mix your lemon juice and apples in a bowl before adding in your cornstarch, sugar and cinnamon. Make sure it's evenly coated.
3. Toss the blueberries in, and then spread the mixture into the baking dish.
4. Get out a bowl and mix baking powder, both flours, sugar and salt together.
5. Cut the margarine and mix it in until it forms a crumbly dough.
6. Stir in the milk and vanilla, and mix well to form a moist dough.
7. Knead with floured hands.
8. Roll it out into a half an inch-thick rectangle.
9. Cut the dough into your favorite shapes using a cookie cutter.
10. Use the remaining scraps to cut more cookies.
11. Place this on top of your apple mixture until it is completely covered, and bake for a half hour before serving.

CONCLUSION

Now you know everything you need to in order to enjoy the benefits of the DASH diet. There's no reason to just deal with hypertension, but remember that even with his dietary change, you will still need any medication prescribed to your by your doctor as well as you'll need to exercise regularly to maintain your health and reap the full benefits. With regular exercise and healthy eating, a dietary approach to stopping hypertension is manageable. Don't let hypertension rule your life. Take back control by first taking back control of your diet.